ER Stories from the Inside

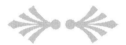

Brian Fleig

If you'd like to connect with me, I can be found at:

Brian@Thenursinginsider.com
http://www.Thenursinginsider.com
http://Facebook.com/Nursinginsider

Dr. Gal D.
Enjoy the stories but please DO NOT read them aloud around me!
George

ER Stories from The Inside
ER Stories: Book one

Copyright ©2019 Brian Fleig

ISBN: 9781794455887

All rights reserved. No part of this book may be reproduced, scanned or transmitted in any forms, digital, audio or printed, without the express written consent by the author.

Table of Contents

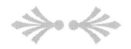

Introduction 7
What is a Code? 10
The ER Team 13
Code in a Very Small California Hospital . . 15
Funny Story from That Same Hospital . . . 19
Burn Victim 22
An Even Worse Burn 25
One Last Burn Victim... For Now 27
38 Caliber Bullet 29
Castle in Nicaragua 32
Weird Arm Scars 34
Movie Character? 36
Bugs Under His Skin 38
Heroin Overdose 41

Weird Flu Patient	43
Security Dude	47
Happy Ending (No, Not that Kind)	49
16-Year-old with Chest Pain	52
My First Trauma	58
Bladder Cancer	61
On a Related Note	64
11-Month-old Girl	67
GHB New Year's Eve Vegas	71
Beware the Truth Serum	75
Harley Dude	77
Hospital Security	79
Another Quick Security Story	83
Oh Shit, Did I Just Do That?	85
Suicide Attempt because of a Phone	88
Another Teen Suicide	90
Kind of an Ethics Question	92
Grapefruit as a Foreign Object	95
A Human Interest Story	96
DEA Agent in Vegas	98
Males are the Biggest Whiners	100
Speaking of Burns	103
Why are Men so Stupid?	108
Drug Seekers: A Huge Frustration	110
Another Major Frustration	114
Suicidal Ideation in the U.S.	116
About the Author	121

Introduction

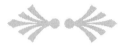

I HAVE TO tell you upfront that, as much as I would like to, I will not be naming hospitals or even hopefully giving enough information for anyone to figure out who is who or where. The reason for that is that patient privacy is so deeply ingrained in all healthcare workers that it just puts the fear into me that someone somewhere might figure out who I'm talking about.

I will start off this storytelling by telling you who I am. I graduated college as a nurse in 1993 so that makes 26 years of Nursing as of writing this. I've been full-time in the emergency room from 2003 to present. Prior to being full-time in the ER I worked almost every place in the hospital. I have worked medical floors in Ortho, Neuro, Urology and Postop. I've done step down ICU, but I will not say that I was ever an ICU nurse. I even floated to a GYN for one night, that was really no fun. I have worked as a hospice nurse, as a home health nurse and I have been on IV teams. Mostly my experience is as a travel nurse rather than a staff nurse and have worked in many states. My first travel contract was actually 10 months after I graduated.

During my time working emergency departments, I have worked four or maybe five Trauma Centers in addition to numerous hospitals where the emergency department was no bigger than 4 beds and just about everything in between. I have worked in eight or nine states and am licensed in even more. One thing I can tell you for sure is that all those years in an emergency room jades you. I know very few if any nurses with more than a year or two in emergency departments who aren't full blown cynics. I am going to try very hard to keep my cynicism out of my writing, but I cannot make any guarantees.

The situations and the stories that I will be telling in this book are not all mine. Most of them are in that I was at least a participant if not the main character. Some of them I was an observer, some of them were detailed stories told to me by co-workers that I missed by not being there that night. Filling in your co-workers is a common practice, sometimes for many days afterwards. Perhaps it's part of coping with it.

We cannot afford to show emotion during it all, the people around us feed off that. If any one of us were visibly falling apart in any way, family members and other patients pick up on that and it escalates. We are human however, and the emotions catch up to us afterwards. Every now and then the emotions are overwhelming.

What you will read here are my opinions and mine alone. While I know that many share my feelings, I will not speak for anyone else much less the collective.

What is a Code?

I THINK A number of the stories I'm going to tell are based on codes, so I better Define a code, as we see a code. And by we, I mean ER staff. A code as you see on television of course involves someone's heart-stopping and ER staff, or whoever, is doing CPR which means chest compressions. Intubating is generally done concurrently with compressions which means inserting a tube down into their lungs and breathing with an AMBU bag followed by a machine called a respirator or ventilator. We just call it a Vent. An Ambu bag is the big round bag connected to the oxygen that someone either plugs into the end of the tube that's into their lungs or it has a mask that clamps over their mouth and nose we use to squeeze oxygen into their lungs. You see it in all the TV shows. We are generally using the Ambu bag during the code and then after the code, assuming we get their heart restarted, is when we hook up the Vent to do the breathing. The third part of a code, and these three parts are equally important, is drugs. At the same time one person is doing chest compressions someone else is forcing oxygen in with the Ambu bag, someone else is obtaining IV (Intra Venous) access so that we can give them drugs to help restart their heart and/or fix the reason the heart stopped in the first place. Those three things, chest compressions, intubation and drugs are the three main tools that we are using in a code.

 Now here is what might confuse people on the outside. Sometimes it's not a code but we call it a code. If someone is, as we say, circling the drain we may refer to that as a code when it's technically not a code because their heart has not stopped. Circling the drain means they're doing really really badly, and their heart will probably be stopping in the very near future. Obviously, we are trying to prevent that from happening and it usually absorbs just as much staff time and stress as a full-blown code.

 Of course, if you've ever watched a code happen on television, whether it's accurate or not accurate, it looks like there's an awful lot more than those three things going on. And of course, there is but those three things are the core interventions that we're doing to bring them back. Everything else is mostly measuring and assessing not actually intervening. I have probably participated in or observed over a hundred codes and honestly, I'm not sure I really remember more than a dozen or so. But those that I remember really do stand out.

The ER Team

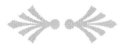

I HAVE WORKED in most areas of a hospital. While I have never been an ICU nurse or an L&D nurse, I have been exposed to those areas enough that I think I can speak to their culture. The one part of the hospital I will not pretend to know the first thing about is the operating room. There are two things I love most about working in the emergency department. One is, of all the places whose culture I can speak for, the ER has the tightest bond between the staff. And by staff, I mean Nurses, CNAs, Techs, Unit Secretaries, Doctors and PA's. We are all equals not one of those job titles is less important than any of the others. If you took away any one of those titles the rest of the staff would suffer, and the efficiency of the entire department would be noticeably less. The bond is truly what I would imagine you would find in a foxhole. I can't describe it any better than that. We have each other's back no matter what and we feel each other's pain, and we generally know what each other is thinking without speaking. I imagine it's much like what they call "the thin blue line".

The other thing I love about the ER is the unpredictability. Nurses who come and try out the ER and cannot cope will probably say it's the unpredictability that drove them away. Floor nurses come on shift and spend up to an hour getting a full report on each and every one of their patients including the most minute details. ER nurses get report from each other that equates to about 60 to 90 seconds per patient. When we get new patients in the door whether they are walk-ins or ambulances we have to figure out what's happening on the fly without a "report". We're doing everything from the moment they arrived. Gathering information, triaging, EKG, starting an IV, drawing blood, hooking up a monitor, talking to family, Etc. when a floor nurse gets a patient all that is already done and I'm not saying they do nothing, they certainly are busy, and they definitely earn their money. But it is a completely different kind of busy and a different atmosphere and it's what I love about the emergency department.

Code in a Very Small California Hospital

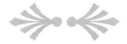

THIS IS A story that was relayed to me by multiple people and the facts in all their stories matched up perfectly, so I feel good about passing it along. It's a story not so much about the subject of the code but about the nurse and the Doctor involved. This was a hospital that was in a town that was so small there were no nurses even living in this town or I should say not enough nurses in this town to staff the whole hospital. The day shift nurses we're locals but the entire night shift, in the ER, was covered by Travelers. This hospital had a 5 Bed ER, a 15 or 20 bed med-surg floor with Telemetry and that was it. No OR, no OB, nothing else at all. The ER travel nurses, of which I was one, would come in to town and work 10 straight shifts, all 12 hours long, and then go home. Three of us covered the entire month. I was there for a total of 9 months or so doing this rotation. Considering that I had 20 days off every month the job and the pay were awesome.

Anyway, I came in for this 10-day stretch and found out that the nurse that worked the previous 10-day stretch had been fired that morning. The night before a guy was brought in by ambulance, CPR in progress. Let me backtrack.

The Doctors that worked in the ER we're also Travelers. They would come for 3 days or 5 days or 7 days or whatever they wanted. They would work straight through around the clock, but they generally were able to sleep at night. Because the hospital was so far out in the country, they had a hard time finding Doctors that would come in at all. It turns out the group who hired the Doctors were telling potential hires that this place was nothing more than a little country Clinic. Well the truth was that it was the only Hospital in a 40- or 50-mile radius which meant anyone who was picked up by ambulance coding in that radius had to come to us first because we were the closest facility. That's a legal thing, closest available facility for medical stabilization. 90% of what we did was treat kids with ear infections, but we actually worked a fairly high number of cardiac arrests because of the fact they had to come to us first. We would stabilize them and then ship them to a bigger hospital, usually by helicopter, that had ICU, surgery, cardiology or whatever specialty was needed.

The Doctor that was on this particular night had started on my last shift before I left my previous stretch. He came in originally wearing a starched white lab coat, a tie and shiny dress shoes. He thought my job was to follow him around with a clipboard and write down his orders. I had to straighten him out on that right away. My job most certainly was not to follow him around. Basically, he thought this was like working in his office and as it turns out his office specialty was ear nose and throat. He had never stepped foot in an ER in his career or it sure appeared that way.

So back to the code. A guy comes in by ambulance in cardiac arrest. CPR is in progress by the ambulance crew and the Doctor freezes. He stands in the corner and cannot talk or do anything else. He had absolutely no idea what to do. So, the nurse intubated the patient. Now back in those days ACLS (Advanced Cardiac Life Support), which is a certification we are all required to maintain, taught intubation. It no longer includes intubation but back then it did. It never made any sense to any of us that we had to learn intubation because intubation is not within the scope of practice for nurses in any state that I'm aware of. Oddly, or perhaps not oddly, paramedics are allowed to intubate. However, the ambulance company in this very small town did not have any paramedics. Luckily in this case the ambulance crew did stick around and help the nurse. They did compressions, ran the Ambu bag and got the IV access.

The nurse intubated the patient and ran the code, which means directed it by giving instructions to the other participants and gave all the medications. The patient lived. The nurse got the patient on a helicopter to another hospital without any input or assistance from the Doctor.

Because intubation was outside her scope of practice per state law and, by extension, hospital policy she was fired in the morning. As the story goes, a month later her California nursing license was revoked for the same reason. Had she not gone outside of her scope of practice that guy would have died in that ER. She basically gave up her ability to make a living to save a guy who may or may not have even made it off the helicopter alive. How fucked up is that?

Funny Story from That Same Hospital

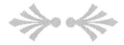

WELL I THINK it's a funny story. This hospital, and I hope I'm not giving away too much as to location, only stayed in business because of two state prisons that were nearby. Now here's a little tidbit for you, both of these state prisons had Million Dollar plus Hospital facilities in house. I had had many conversations with CO's (correction officers) and facility nurses by phone. One of the nurses once told me that they had a full-time around the clock Doctor and Psychiatrist on staff who was on call. They were making some ridiculous amount of money to be on call somewhere in the quarter million dollars a year range. When they would call the psychiatrist or the Doctor at night the response, 100% of the time, was to send the patient to the hospital. That meant us. So, if you live in California this is a very small example of where your tax dollars go.

    We would get a lot of inmates; each inmate would come with two CO's. One would be the hands-on guy managing the cuffs and chains and the other would stand back at a distance because he was carrying the gun. When our little tiny Hospital filled up with inmates this made for an awful lot of CO's standing around, each of them seeming to come with a 2'x2' square soft sided lunch cooler. We got all sorts of different complaints from the inmates, complaint meaning the reason they were there. One of the big complaints from inmates was facial Trauma from fights. One particular night a guy comes in with particularly serious facial trauma, not trauma center serious trauma but definitely ruined his entire month facial trauma. This guy was really messed up. We CAT scanned his skull and facial bones, but I don't recall if he had any fractures.

    Normally the CO's would not tell us any backstories of inmates, they are not supposed to. Every once in a while, though they would let something out that would be important for us to know. I would always ask anyway because I was curious and sometimes, they would open up. Well on this guy on this night with a little bit worse than usual facial trauma I asked. The answer was he was being escorted to solitary confinement. They probably did not use the term solitary confinement but that was my assumption that that's what their terminology meant. On his way to solitary confinement his CO escorts warned him about a dangerous set of steel steps going down. They told him to be careful these steps are dangerous, but he tripped and fell down the steps in spite of the warning. Then he walked back up the steps and fell down the steps again. They told me this with an absolutely straight face, so I just stared at them for a minute with a smirk on my face because I knew there was more to it. Then the rest of the story came out.

He had gaslighted one of the CO'S. What is gas-lighting you ask? Well one of the inmates' hobbies, apparently, is to collect their own waste in a receptacle. Think coffee mug or coffee can or something like that. We are talking feces, urine, spit, blood. If the mixture comes out too thick, they can thin it out with a little water. What they do with this delicious soup is to throw it in someone's face, I assume an enemy's face. This guy's mistake was throwing it in a CO's face. Maybe he wanted to spend some time in solitary. Doesn't that sound like a fun place to work?

Burn Victim

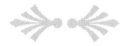

I was working at a level 1 Trauma Center on the West Coast or near the West Coast. This particular place separated the trauma ER and the pediatric ER from the adult medical ER. They were three separate physical places in two different buildings. At the time I worked there they were the second busiest ER and the fourth busiest Trauma Center in the country, or maybe it was the other way around. Strangely, all burn victims came to the adult medical ER not to the trauma ER. This Trauma Center had an in-house Burn Unit so when we got a burn patient in the ER, we would call the burn center and one or two Burn Center nurses would come down to the ER to take over treatment after the initial intake.

After having been assigned to one relatively minor burn patient I Started a conversation with one of the burn center nurses. As a result of that conversation I decided I wanted to get ABLS (Advanced Burn Life Support). It had absolutely nothing to do with how good-looking and single the burn center nurse was. It was all about being the first ER nurse at that hospital that had that certification which sounded pretty cool. I asked the director of the ER if the hospital would pay the $250 for the certification class and was told no. I did the only logical thing and paid for the class out-of-pocket and again it had absolutely nothing to do with how good-looking and single this nurse was so get that out of your head.

A month or so after the class we got a real burn patient. It was not my patient, but I wandered over there to help and hopefully apply some of what I had learned. In this and every other ER I've worked in whenever a difficult patient comes in you will have lots of help. In some cases, if it's a larger ER with a lot of staff, there will be so much help in the room there won't be enough space for everyone. That was the case with this burn patient. When I wandered over to help the room was already full, but I was determined to apply my new certification.

The room was full, so I approached the patient's feet because that was the only spot without a nurse. The big thing with any new patient of this type whether it's trauma, heart attack or especially in the case of a burn is you want to get all their clothes off. I approached her feet and started pulling off her socks. Unfortunately for me, and even more so for her, the socks came right off right along with the skin of her feet. We call that degloving and I believe her entire body degloved as all of her clothes were removed. I remember that it turned out that she had second and third-degree Burns over a massive part of her body probably 70% or more. She did not live which was probably the best thing that could have happened for her. You may think that sounds cold but when you're in the middle of it that's the reality. Talk to a burn center nurse if you ever get a chance and ask what the rehab and healing process looks like.

 Just to put closure on this particular story we found out later that she was homeless and living in a small homemade tent on a sidewalk. She had a small kerosene or propane powered space heater in her tent which started the tent on fire. There were numerous cops and fire personnel there in the ER and one or two of them talked like they suspected someone set the fire on purpose. In the end though that possibility was never pursued, that I know of. None of us ever even found out what her name was, and I seriously doubt the cops or coroner could get any finger prints for ID.

 A week or so after that the ER director decided that the hospital would pay for the entire staff to go through ABLS certification on a volunteer basis. Of course, I was never reimbursed but I didn't care. I never saw that burn center nurse again by the way.

An Even Worse Burn

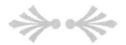

SOMETIME AFTER THE previous burn patient, I think it was a few months, we got an even worse burn patient in the same ER. This one was a mid-20s female, as far as we could tell. She had third-degree Burns over 90% of her body if not 100%. In this case I was out in the hallway watching because the room had already filled up with help. I was a little glad to be out in the hallway for this one because she had so much flesh burned away that people were trying to put IV needles into veins that were completely exposed. Think of a thigh with nothing left but exposed veins and arteries right there out in the open. On a side note, what people don't realize about surviving a severe burn is the months and months of extremely painful healing it takes. From what I have been told the words extremely painful don't do it justice.

One of the nurses in the room had just finished her first TNCC certification. It stands for Trauma Nurse Core Course. The biggest thing you need to know about TNCC is that they teach you to physically and visually inspect the entire body starting at the top of the head all the way to the feet. What I mean by this is you are literally putting both hands on and feeling for foreign bodies, crunchy bones or anything else out of place front and back, head to foot. So, this nurse who had just finished her first TNCC certification was standing at the Patients head and started doing the exam. I wondered to myself what made her think to do that and just figured, well she just learned it so why not.

Well she didn't even get past the head because one of the fingers of her gloved hands slid right through the skull into the victim's brain. This was obviously unexpected, and I could see by her face that it freaked her out a little bit or maybe a lot of bit. So long story short, it turns out that the fire was set by her boyfriend to hide the fact he had murdered her with one or more hammer strikes to the head. Think of the round head of a carpenter's Hammer hitting your head so hard that it drives that piece of skull into your brain. Oh, by the way, she was also pregnant which some surmised was the cause of the fight. She did not live and neither did the baby.

One Last Burn Victim... For Now

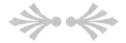

SAME HOSPITAL SAME section of the ER one bed over from where the female murder victim laid. An ambulance comes in with an apparently 30 something year old Japanese male who had doused himself with gasoline at a gas station and set himself on fire. Just so you know, we never know the background stories or the reasons for things like this usually until much later. We wouldn't know it at all except for being told by firemen on the scene or cops. This was another one that I was out in the hallway because I was too slow getting there which was perfectly fine by me. By this time, I had figured out that being a burn nurse was not in my future and neither was dating one.

Well this was another one that was burned second and third degree over 80 to 100% of his body. His clothes were melted into his flesh so thoroughly that there was no way of separating him from his clothes. His backstory was that he had a wife and kids who were all Japanese and he owned a business. Apparently, his business was doing poorly, I have no idea how poorly, but poorly enough that he thought it was his duty to kill himself. Whoever I heard telling this story said that he was yelling to the people in the gas station something about being a failure.

The smell of gasoline in the department was so bad we had to smell it for the entire rest of the shift. The ambulance crew that brought him in spent hours in our ambulance bay trying to clean the gasoline and charred people smell out of the back of the ambulance. My main memory of that case was standing there thinking to myself it's bad enough that you would choose to kill yourself for a financial problem ok but why anyone would choose to do it the way he did was beyond me.

38 Caliber Bullet

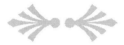

OKAY SO FOR this story I will divulge the location. It was UMC in Las Vegas otherwise known as University Medical Center. It is a level 1 Trauma Center. We would get a fair number of gunshot victims in the medical ER that should have gone to the Trauma ER. The medical ER faced the street and was most visible to the public while the Trauma ER was around back in a different building. The result was that people that drove their buddy to the ER would just pull up to the front door where it said emergency. Now I have to admit that in the year I was there I only saw probably 4 or 5 or gunshot victims. The funny thing to me was that each and every gunshot victim that I saw were driven up to the door by their homies and basically dumped. They would beep the horn then bail out and run or just shove the victim out onto the sidewalk and drive away. In one case the guy that was shot actually drove himself up to the door and crawled to the door or maybe people standing outside smoking brought him to our attention. His car was full of bullet holes.

What surprised me about The Gunshot victims that I did see was not in a single case was there any visible external blood. Being a medical ER and not the trauma ER all we did was start IVs, start fluids running, take their Vital Signs and ship them over to the trauma department. I don't know how many of them lived although each and every one of them had bullet wounds in their torso. Each and every one of them however was alive when we got them to the trauma bay.

Okay so now about the 38-caliber bullet. This actually happened to me one night when I was at UMC in what we called the Fast Track. It was six or eight beds that were supposed to be fast in and out stuff that did not need time consuming workups, IV's or cardiac monitors. This particular night one of the guys that came in was there because he had a 38-caliber bullet pressing on his skin from the inside. It was clearly visible when he pointed it out on his left hip. The bullet was trying to break itself out through his skin. Of course, I had to ask him how the hell it got there. He laughed and said he had been shot in the opposite hip, I believe he said it had been 6 months before that. I said, so wait a minute you were shot in the other hip in the bullet came all the way through to this hip? He said, "yes and it missed everything on the way through". When it originally happened, the Doctor had told him it was not worth surgically removing because it was not endangering anything. I asked him how the hell does a bullet go in one hip all the way through to the other hip and missed the bladder and all the major blood vessels. He laughed again and said, "it did".

He showed me the scar on his other hip and sure enough it was there and sure enough it looked like it was appropriate to the age that he said it was. He said that the bullet was not pressing against the skin to come out originally but over time it had worked its way to where it was bothering him because of rubbing on the skin trying to break out. The PA that was running that department that night gave him a little shot of Lidocaine at the site and with a scalpel made a really small slice and pulled out a 38-caliber slug. He got a dose of antibiotics by mouth and a prescription for more to take home with him.

Castle in Nicaragua

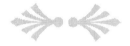

THIS STORY TAKES me all the way back to college. I believe it was fall of 1992, my first semester. The story is about someone who was in the class ahead of me, so he was in his third semester. The story is also hearsay; however, it comes from a very reliable source. One of my classmates worked part-time in the hospital where this happened, and it was a very very small Hospital. You might remember if you were alive sometime around 1990 our military was assaulting a castle in Nicaragua. They were blasting rock music at ridiculously high volumes and cutting off supplies from going into the castle. They were trying to get Manuel Noriega to come out so he could be arrested.

Back to the story. the guy that I'm talking about was in his third semester of nursing school. This particular day he was doing clinical in the PACU (Post Anesthesia Care Unit) of this very small Hospital. That's where you go after surgery to gradually wake up and let the anesthesia wear off while they monitor you. As the Story goes, he was at the bedside of a female patient who was really groggy just coming out of anesthesia and apparently confused. She asked him, because he was the first person she saw, "where am I?". His response to her was "you are in a castle in Nicaragua". She screamed at the top of her lungs bringing Hospital staff to the bedside. I have no idea how he explained her screaming to the staff, but I bet her anesthesia wore off really quick.

Somehow, miraculously, he avoided being kicked out of the program. In fact, two years later he ended up being my charge nurse for one night at Highland Hospital in Rochester NY which I really hated. I didn't like him very much completely unrelated to that story.

Weird Arm Scars

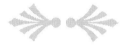

WE ARE BACK in California again and we have a state inmate in an ER bed. I don't remember what this guy's story was and it doesn't really matter, I can't even remember why he was there in the ER. While I was taking his blood pressure, I noticed some really weird scars on his arm. Now I remember back to high school when some kids / idiots would brag about what they called Bowl Burns. What they did was they would take a pot pipe otherwise known as a bowl and heat the top edge of it up with a lighter and then use it to Brand themselves, usually on the forearms. Apparently, it was some sort of badge of honor, I don't know.

This inmate who was probably in his forties, give or take, had what looked like they might have been bowl burns on one forearm. Of course, I had to ask, what the scars were about, I think there were five or six of them. He looked me right in the eye and with an absolute dead pan voice told me they were 45 caliber bullet wounds. I asked him who would shoot you in the arm and his reply was he had done it himself. He did admit to being Stoned on something at the time and when I asked him why he would do that he responded that he was trying to kill himself.

I took half a minute or so to digest this. I cannot even begin to imagine how much it would hurt to shoot yourself at point-blank range with a 45-caliber bullet five or six times. I can't even begin to imagine what drug you could take that would leave you awake enough to do that and yet give you enough pain control that would allow you to do it over and over and over. I looked over at the CO who was just grinning, and I asked the guy, well how did that work out for you? Again, he looked right at me and with a flat deadpan monotone voice said, "not very well". The CO had to leave the room because he was about to burst out laughing.

One of my observations after dealing with a lot of inmates was that there were very few intelligent inmates.

Movie Character?

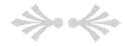

SAME HOSPITAL, DIFFERENT inmate, same prison. This guy comes in, I think it was on Christmas with a dislocated shoulder. It was a legit dislocated shoulder, so we did what we call a conscious sedation and put his shoulder back in place. Actually, nowadays we have to call it a moderate sedation or some nonsense. They had to change the terminology for some legal ridiculousness. Conscious sedation is done with a drug that mostly knocks you out. Which drug we use depends on the Doctor that's doing it. Different Doctors have different preferences. The bottom line is there are probably four or five different drugs that we could potentially use, none of which I ever associated with getting high.

It wasn't maybe three or four minutes later the Doctor had walked away, I had to stand next to the bed watching the monitor until the guy came out of the Sedation, and his shoulder was back out of place. So, we got to do it all over again. Yay. 5 minutes after that we were doing it a third time. This time as I'm watching the monitor, and I'm watching him and sure enough I caught him popping his shoulder out deliberately. I never would have guessed it was even possible, but I watched him do it. He was skinny enough that we sure didn't need an x-ray to see all kinds of displacement.

When I told the doc what I saw he was pissed, and I wasn't very happy about it either. The doc comes back in the room, and he's a no-nonsense kind of guy. I really liked this Doc, and he tells the guy well you're so good at popping your shoulder out you can damn well pop it back in. He tried to deny it for a couple minutes then he complained about it for a couple more minutes then he popped his own shoulder back in and got discharged. I didn't see him get it back in but given that he was handcuffed to the stretcher he sure didn't slam his shoulder against any walls. And he didn't yell either. The CO was equally amazed, and he said well sometimes these guys will do anything just to get a little holiday high. So, I guess that scene in Lethal Weapon where Mel Gibson pops his shoulder back in is maybe not so fake after all.

Bugs Under His Skin

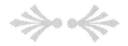

BACK IN NEVADA now working at a fairly big hospital. 99% of nursing shifts start at 7 p.m. if they are 12-hour shifts. So, I would walk in this place at 6:30 because they actually had a really nice break room and it was pleasant to go in there with your co-workers and kind of get your game face on before the shift. Most break rooms are actually way too small and really crappy but this one was nice. Every day I walked in I would come in through the ambulance bay because there's no way I was going to walk through a hundred pissed off people in the lobby while wearing scrubs making a verbal target of myself. That would be like walking across a driving range at the golf course with a target on your head. On the way to the break room I would always stop at a computer and check the lobby to see how many people were out there and it was never less than 75 and sometimes it was up to a hundred. The average wait time at any Hospital in Las Vegas at that time was anywhere from 8 to 12 hours in the lobby.

What was really cool about this particular computer system was you could sort it based on patient name, how long they had been there, or their complaint which is the reason they were there. I would sort it by complaint and on any given day there were between 10 and 20 spider bites listed as complaints. Complaints of spider bites never turned out to be spider bites. They were open sores from crystal meth 100% of the time. I don't know if it's the same now in fact I haven't seen any one that had taken crystal meth in quite a while. We could always tell who they were because they were tweaking. Their body was constantly twitching so we called them tweakers. The way crystal meth was made, at least in those days, was to mix the active ingredient heavily with Drano or an equally nasty filler. I actually got that information from a DEA agent at that same Hospital who was there with a prisoner one time.

The problem with using Drano as a filler and then having people snort it is that your body cannot process Drano. It is not leaving your body via the liver or the kidneys or your bowels which is how your body gets rid of things. The only thing left is for it to work its way out through your skin, literally. I read that in a magazine article. Crystal meth was insanely popular in those days. I think I've maybe seen only one tweaker in The Last 5 Years come to think of it. Either that drug fell out of favor or it's being manufactured differently now.

So, this guy is in his thirties or forties and he just comes off as a white-collar professional to me. He strikes me as a pretty smart guy who probably has a bachelor's or master's degree in something. Maybe he works in an office maybe he's even in some sort of science related job. That was the impression he gave me. This guy spent 45 minutes telling me how he had bugs crawling under his skin which was also a pretty common complaint with tweakers. He even went as far as to tell me that he cut out a small square patch of his skin and put it under a microscope and could see the bugs moving under the microscope. He said I'll go home and get you the slide and bring it in. I have to admit he almost had me convinced that he might have had something. Of course, if he was really that convinced, he should have brought the slide with him, not that we have microscopes in the ER. We don't. I think he got a shot of Ativan or something else to offset the meth and then went home.

Heroin Overdose

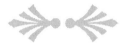

HEROIN OVERDOSES SEEM to come in spurts depending on where you are geographically, I suppose. Virtually anyone that comes into the ER that's less than 60 years old and unresponsive is going to most likely get a dose of IV Narcan. You might have heard about it on the television news that fire departments and police are carrying Narcan now because of the so-called opioid epidemic. I'm not sure what form they're giving it in possibly an aerosol spray because that would work very quickly. It can also be given IM or intramuscularly which means a shot. We give it IV or intravenously because it works almost instantaneously. You can take a full-blown heroin (Or any other opioid) overdose patient who is barely breathing (because that's what opioids do), shoot a milligram or even a half a milligram of Narcan into his vein and he's going to be wide awake in seconds and really pissed off. They're generally very angry with us because we just stole their high that they paid for.

If the Narcan does not wake them up, then we know it's not an opioid problem. It's very useful to try Narcan first because there are no negative effects from it and it's fast. One of my favorite ER Doctors was at a hospital outside of Las Vegas. We got a lot of heroin addicts at that particular Hospital. His favorite trick was to discharge them, once we made sure they were stable, but just before discharge we would give them two mg of Narcan IM in a shot. Any drug given into a muscle in the form of a shot takes longer before it works, unlike given via the IV, however it lasts much longer. We're talking probably hours depending on the drug and the person. Yes, I will admit to getting much satisfaction out of sitting at the ER desk thinking that that guy we just sent home is going to rush to his dealer and shoot another dose of heroin as quick as he can but it ain't going to do him any good. Not for at least 2 or 3 hours. That Narcan in his system is going to cancel out that heroin until the Narcan wears off. You're welcome.

Weird Flu Patient

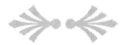

I THINK IT was my very first shift in the ER working at a particular Hospital in Las Vegas. I was there through a local staffing agency. Ten or twenty minutes before the end of my shift, I get an ambulance. Dammit, that's the last thing any nurse wants minutes before shift change. The guy is 40-45 years old give or take a couple years. The ambulance crew says he lived in a nice house and he was alone in the house. The report from the ambulance crew was that when they arrived on scene there was vomit all over the house and the guy. He was wandering around aimlessly and refused to speak to them. Now drug addicts of all ages in Las Vegas were extremely common and every indication was that this guy was just another stoned druggy.

He was able to get himself off the ambulance gurney and walk into the room which was just another indicator that he wasn't actually sick, other than vomiting obviously, but that he was probably just high. By the way when an ER nurse uses the word sick, they're talking dangerously ill. Not like oh your kid is too sick to go to school, that's not sick to us. Sick is your blood pressure is crashing, your heart is palpitating, you're sweating buckets, you're having a stroke, Etc. I'm not minimizing how miserable it is to "feel sick', it happens to me too but it's not "sick" by ER standards.

I'm not taking my kids to an ER unless he presents to me his detached finger in a baggie. If it's just dangling but still attached, well that's why God gave us duct tape.

So, I worked this guy up in my last few minutes. I got him undressed and in to a hospital gown, took his blood pressure, started an IV and drew blood for lab and recorded report from the ambulance crew because I could not get any information from the guy. That's basically what's known as a triage. The ambulance crew had already checked his blood sugar and it was okay.

I came back in that night at 7 p.m. and found out from the nurse that I had passed that guy off to that within an hour after I left, he had gone to the ICU because his blood pressure started crashing. It turns out he tested positive for the flu. Not your kid stays home sick with flu symptoms but the actual flu. I have seen a lot of people with the actual flu over the years and he is by far the sickest one that I have seen and the only one that came close to death because of the flu. Of course, I don't know if he had some sort of underlying medical problem that made the flu worse in his case. So of course, I felt guilty because I had written him off as a druggie but given the signs that I saw and the few minutes that I had with him I don't think I did anything wrong, but I did feel guilty regardless.

I worked the rest of that night and left and went back to my hotel room. I just arrived in Vegas that week or the week before and I was staying in an extended stay hotel room. I had sprung the extra cost and got the room that actually had a separate bedroom, So I actually had basically two rooms that were connected one was the standard full-sized refrigerator, bathroom, sink, couch, TV and then the next room had a bed, TV and a chair.

I don't think I was back in the room more than an hour when I started feeling sick. Lucky for me I was not scheduled that night and within an hour of starting to feel sick I found that I could not talk. My mental capacity was normal, and I could certainly formulate thoughts, but I absolutely could not speak them out loud. I thought about calling someone, but I didn't for two reasons, one I didn't know anyone in Las Vegas and two I literally could not speak. Also lucky for me, I had a full 28 pack of bottled water in my room. So, I gathered an armload of bottled water put it next to the bed along with a garbage can to throw up in and my cell phone just in case I needed 911. Because I figured the guy's blood pressure had crashed because he was hypovolemic (dehydrated) I was determined to avoid my condition deteriorating to what his was, but I now understood why he refused to talk to us.

It took me three days of crawling between the bed and the bathroom in that hotel room before I could stand up and walk out the door and breathe fresh air again, but I never had to call 911 because I kept myself hydrated. That was the only time in 26 years that I ever brought anything home from the hospital other than the sniffles and I'm not even sure about the sniffles.

Security Dude

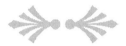

ANOTHER LAS VEGAS story. There were three things that we got in the ER in Las Vegas more than any other city I have worked. They were psych patients, drunks, and druggies. Very often those three things were all rolled into one person. We used a lot of restraints in Las Vegas both physical and chemical. In the physical restraint department, we used both soft restraints and leather restraints. This one particular hospital that I work at had a security guard that work nights that I kid you not was six foot six maybe six foot seven and probably 300 lb. His body fat percentage was less than 10%, this guy was a wall of muscle. If that was not enough, he was ex-military. I don't know exactly what he did in the military, but the stories were that he was special forces. He was as nice as anyone you would want to meet but I'm guessing he may have been the most dangerous human I have ever met.

When we had someone, whose behavior was bad enough that we needed to use leather restraints we would call this guy. Assuming the behavior was due to a psych problem and the patient was able to comprehend what was happening around him, vs being stoned or drunk, just the sight of this guy would very often preclude the need for restraints. I'm not a small guy but I never had that kind of effect on people and it sure was nice having that guy around.

Happy Ending (No, Not that Kind)

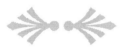

OKAY SO THIS certainly was not happy for the patient, but it was not sad for the staff. This is another Hospital in Las Vegas. This particular night 90% of the staff happened to be male and one of our patients, which was not uncommon in Las Vegas, was a professional stripper. This particular stripper was also very high on something. I don't think any of us knew what or at least I don't remember what. I don't even remember why she was in the hospital, but she wasn't really sick I think she was probably there because she acted like a wackadoodle and someone called an ambulance and anything that nobody else can explain or handle comes to the emergency room. In fact, ironically, now days cops bring all drunks to the emergency room before they are allowed to go to jail. They say its jail policy that drunks need to have medical clearance because supposedly one time long ago some drunk died in a jail cell. That's actually not hard to believe but I personally think the cops prefer to dump them on the ER because then they don't have to deal with them. Sometimes they sit there and wait for them to be medically cleared and then take them to jail and then sometimes they just dump them and leave them after writing them an appearance ticket. In fact, a lot of times cops will order an ambulance crew to take the drunk to the hospital because they don't want the drunk throwing up in the police car. Ask any ambulance people in any City if that happens.

So anyway, however she got there and whatever reason she was there for, she was there. The less than sad thing for the staff and the less than happy thing for the patient was that she had no idea where she was or who she was or what year it was or anything else that you and I take for granted. And apparently, having no mental capacity to reason she reverted to base instincts. She absolutely refused to keep her gown on, and she absolutely refused to stay under the sheet or in the bed for that matter. Every 15 minutes or so she was up naked as the day she was born walking around the ER. So being the good nurses that we were we would give her 2 or 3 minutes to walk around so that we could assess her ability to walk a straight line of course and then we would put her back in bed and cover her back up with the sheet. 15 minutes later, rinse and repeat. Now had this been a little old lady who was at risk for falling we would have most likely used soft restraints to keep her in the bed. Had this been a male stripper he would have been securely restrained in bed. For his own safety of course.

She was perfectly steady on her feet and there's a big national move, and has been for a long time, to limit the use of restraints. So naked girl, steady on her feet walking around the ER, restraints are bad, I have had worse shifts.

16-Year-old with Chest Pain

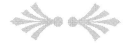

I WAS WORKING in a medium sized hospital in Northern Nevada. This hospital had some services available to it, but it did not have Cardiology on the weekends. This kid comes in that is 16 years old and he has chest pain. Now our standard treatment for anyone that walks in and says they have chest pain is to run them through all the cardiac tests. Honestly, my attitude towards young people with chest pain and I'm talking teens and twenties and even 30s is I think they're being sissies. And I think most other healthcare workers think the same thing. Because you're just not going to have a heart attack in your teens or twenties or thirties. Now that being said it does happen but it's so rare that it's kind of ridiculous.

This kid's story was that he has a job after school at McDonald's and he was riding his bike home, this is 9 or 10 at night, and he started feeling chest pain. I started to take the kid seriously because he seemed like a straight-up kid. He wasn't your typical, I'm going to whine about everything, and I don't believe in taking any responsibility for myself. His mother came in a few minutes after he got there which was good because technically, we need a parent there anyway for permission to treat. Mom actually was just as impressive as the kid in terms of down to earth normal stand-up kind of people. I deliberately sent mom out of the room at one point so that I could talk to the kid by himself just for a minute. I think I told her to go out to registration and double-check paperwork or something. While she was gone, I asked the kid if he had taken any drugs. I gave him my usual speech, "I don't care if you took anything, but we really need to know what you took so that we can treat you correctly".

The kid denied it flat out. When Mom came back, I asked her in front of the kid if she thought there was any possibility that he had taken any drugs. She said no way. between how they both came off is stand up people and their comfortable relationship with each other I absolutely believed them both. At this point, and the drug questioning only took the first three or four minutes, I started hooking up the monitor on the wall to the kid. When I hooked up the final wire of the monitor, I glanced back over my shoulder at the monitor then look back at the kid and then thought to myself holy shit what did I just see. So, I looked back around at the monitor and saw v-tach without the tach. In other words, every Beat was a ventricular beat, but it was a normal rate where that rhythm is normally very fast.

To give that a little perspective, v-tach is a potentially life-threatening rhythm. It is possible to have a short run of v-tach and not have any symptoms of it, but this kid was running non-stop v-tach without the tach. I immediately went to get the EKG machine with shows heart rhythms in much finer detail than the monitor on the wall. Hooked him up, ran the EKG and handed the result to the doctor. He must have stared at that thing, circled beats and wrote little notes for a half an hour while he scratched his head. Meanwhile the kid had no symptoms, no shortness of breath, no sweating, but still had mild pain. So, the pain and possibly the bad heart rhythm apparently was triggered by stressing himself physically.

Immediately after handing the EKG to the doctor I started putting in an IV so that I could draw blood and we would have venous access in case we needed to give him medications. Standard stuff. While I was getting ready to put an IV in his arm his mother told me that the kid's father would pass out when anyone poked him with a needle. I looked at her and smiled and thought to myself that's not the kind of thing that's genetic. This kid has been here now for 15 or 20 minutes and he is impressing me more and more with how mature he is. I take his arm in my left hand and I put the IV into a vein with my right hand. His eyes immediately roll into the back of his head and his cardiac rhythm flatlines. And to this day I still have a copy of that strip showing V-Tach without attack going to Flatline and after about 10 to 15 seconds going back to V-Tach without the tach. I was stunned at this point and did not even think to call for help I'm just kind of holding my breath and lucky for the kid it was only 10 or 15 seconds long and then he's back to normal. In 26 years of putting IVs in people I have never seen anything even remotely like that.

Meanwhile, the doctor calls another doctor and they're both staring at the EKG and now I have two or three follow-up printouts thinking maybe the first one was a fluke. Both doctors are scratching their head and they're on the phone with a cardiologist. after faxing a copy of the EKG to the cardiologist at his house, the cardiologist says, "He has probably had this condition since he was born and is only now symptomatic for it so send him home and I will see him in my office on Monday". At this point we're waiting for lab results from the blood and the doctor is still scratching his head. Nobody has an answer for what could be causing this.

30 or so minutes later all the lab results are in and everything is normal, now the doctor is really scratching his head. He was expecting, if not hoping, that something would be off. If something had been off on in his lab results it would have been kind of nice because it would have at least led down the road towards an explanation. Finally, after probably 2 hours the kids still has no further complaints of shortness of breath or anything you would expect from having a heart problem except for ongoing mild chest pain, but he is still running this weird ventricular rhythm. The doc decides he is not going to send the kid home because he has a weird rhythm that's unexplainable and he's having chest pain. He agrees it's probably congenital and he was probably born with it, but he's here now on Friday night having chest pain.

We transfer the kid by ambulance to a hospital across town that has a cardiologist on call available to see him that night. This is about 10 or 11 at night. At 6 the next morning before we leave at 7 one of us calls the other hospital to find out what happened with this kid because we are all curious. It turns out we didn't get any details of the case, but we did find out they followed up our work up with their own work up and sent the kid to the OR to have a pacemaker placed. They thought it was enough of an emergency that they did it that night which means they had to call in the entire OR crew from home.

That was one of the stranger cases I've ever been associated with and it was a reminder that you can laugh at people for being sissies all you want but you still better check.

My First Trauma

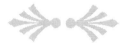

I WAS WORKING at a Trauma Center somewhere in New Hampshire, and I hope that doesn't give away which hospital it was. Then again it probably doesn't matter. In comes this kid, I don't remember how old he was 15 to 17 or somewhere in there. His upper lip was dangling by nothing but a thread of skin at each end of the lip. Otherwise, it was completely separated from his face.

His story was somewhat interesting. He was at one of those teenage parties next to a River out in the woods that involved a bonfire and of course a keg of beer. Since he was too young to drink, I didn't believe him that there could be beer at a party full of teenagers. I mean what teenager would do that? At any rate there he was at a party with a bunch of teenagers, a bunch of beer and a bonfire and apparently some cans of spray paint. Somebody had thrown a can of spray paint into the bonfire because it seems like a cool thing to do.

This particular party going teenager was not pleased with how long it was taking for this can of spray paint to explode in the fire. So naturally, he approached the fire and looked down at the can of spray paint expecting to find out why it was taking so long to explode. Either to mock him or to respond to his unspoken question it was at that moment the can exploded. The base of the can, that little ridge around the bottom, came shooting straight up and hit him perfectly around the mouth. He's lucky it didn't do more damage than it did, but it almost completely cut his upper lip away from his face.

Lucky me, I got to hold the suction while the doctor sewed his lip back on his face. as I'm standing behind the stretcher above the kid's head holding the suction and watching him suture, I'm asking myself why he is sewing his lip to his gums. Literally the sutures were going through the kids gum just above and in between his teeth. I did not ask this question out loud, I was saving it for later, but while I was watching it occurred to me. Where else is he going to sew it to, there's nothing else there?

Since then I have worked other traumas involving dangling body parts. It was dangling body parts that convinced me that I really would prefer not to work trauma. It didn't gross me out or make me faint or any of those things. I was always able to do my job without hesitation or squeamishness, but I had the Epiphany that I just don't need to see dangling body parts to feel like my life was complete. Since I had the trauma nurse certification the manager of every new ER that I worked in as a traveler offered to assign me to the trauma room. My response was always I will do it if I have to, but I would prefer not to and surprisingly nobody ever tried to force me to work in the trauma room. That made me happy.

Bladder Cancer

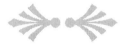

OKAY SO THIS is actually a hospice story not an ER story. This was in a hospice residence in Florida. Most hospices, that I know of, have residences that act as an inpatient setting. The point of hospice is so that you can spend your last days comfortably at home in familiar and comfortable surroundings rather than in a hospital full of beeps, buzzes and strangers interrupting your sleep. The great part about hospice is it they typically will get you whatever kind of medical equipment that you need in your house. This includes hospital beds, walkers, oxygen setups or whatever else you might need. However, even with that level of assistance sometimes people get to a point where their family just cannot keep up with their needs, so they end up in the hospice residence where there is full time nursing care.

One particular guy was 70-plus years old and had end-stage bladder cancer. At the time I was a full-time call nurse, but I happened to be in the residence this particular Saturday afternoon. There was also a couple of field staff in the residence at the time in addition to the regular residence staff. We were helping out with this guy because he was actively bleeding extensively from his bladder. I can still picture it today four of us at his bedside rolling him back and forth changing the absorbent pads under him for this bleeding. We were literally changing his pads almost as fast as we could roll him back and forth from side to side. He was unconscious at the time.

As we often did in the hospice business, we were trying to guess how long he had to live. It sounds cold and crass, but we did not do it because we found people dying to be entertaining. We did it because estimating how long people had to live was somewhat of a valuable skill when you work for hospice. Almost without exception, when you worked in the field, family would ask you that question. "How long do you think he or she has left?" so, it was a skill that we all tended to work on, but no one ever actually got it right, at least not consistently. Occasionally we'd get one right but it's just not something that you can apply science to because everyone is different. That particular day all four of us were making guesses ranging from hours to one or two days.

As it turns out, all four of us could not have been more wrong. This guy fooled all of us and walked out of there 6 months later to rent his own apartment. In fact, I remember seeing a Christmas card from the guy 6 months after he moved out of the hospice residence. Ironically around that same time. I had a home health patient who also had bladder cancer although he did not yet have a terminal prognosis. He told me that he was trying to set up a trip to Germany where they had surgically implanted synthetic bladders. Of course, they had not been FDA-approved in the US because the U.S. is often behind on medical procedures and products thanks to the FDA. I know they SAY it's for our safety, and I am sure sometimes it is, but I can't help but wonder how many FDA approvals are dependent on cash payments. I don't know if that guy ever made it to Germany or not, I never saw him again after that visit.

On a Related Note

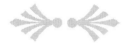

I APOLOGIZE BUT I have one more non-ER story. That last story about the bladder cancer reminded me of this. I was working at a City Hospital in New York not New York City, upstate New York. This was in sometime in the late 90s and I was working on a med-surg floor. One night around midnight the charge nurse tells me there's a patient coming in that I have to admit which is never fun as a nurse, the admission paperwork that is. As it turns out it wasn't bad because the story made up for the ridiculous paperwork.

It was roughly 1 or 2 in the morning when this lady comes in by ambulance directly to the med-surg floor which is extremely unusual. She was unresponsive which means unconscious in this case. Her husband was with her. He was roughly about 70 so and i'm assuming she was about the same age. He told me the story. He had just flown her into the airport by private jet from Mexico. She had been diagnosed as terminal two or three years before that by her doctor in New York, and I don't even remember what the disease was. Her New York doctor told the husband and the patient that there was nothing more that could be done so the husband started doing research. Bear in mind this was in the very early days of the World Wide Web, so I doubt that he got any information from the internet. He may have gotten the information directly from his doctor, I don't know.

At any rate, when he heard there was nothing more that could be done here, he flew his wife to Mexico, again by private jet. She received treatments in Mexico that were not yet approved in the US. It did not cure her, but she did live another two or three years. The downside I suppose was I believe she had to spend those final Years in Mexico for ongoing treatment. Having lost a wife to cancer myself I can tell you that I would have given everything I had to get two or three more years. Our wonderful FDA strikes again.

One of the first strikes that I worked on was down just outside of New York City. Strikes are like travel assignments to the extreme, every single nurse you work with is a travel nurse just like you. On that strike I met a nurse from Birmingham Alabama. She was anxious to work in New York because being from Alabama everyone assumed that New York was the mecca for cutting edge in healthcare. Well she was sorely disappointed. She told me one day that we were five to ten years behind where they were in Birmingham. That was 1999 and she described to me their bedside computer charting system. We did not even have computers in the nurse's station much less at bedside, we were still charting on paper. In fact, we didn't go to computerized charting until well into the 2000s at least not on a broad scale. In fact, I remember working at a fairly large Hospital in Las Vegas in the ER in 2004 and still doing everything on paper, we didn't have a computer anywhere in sight. So, in summary, New York is not the cutting edge of much of anything.

11-Month-old Girl

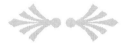

I WAS WORKING in a medium sized Hospital in Las Vegas many years ago and we got a radio call from a helicopter. Actually, I think it was a phone call because this particular ER did not have a radio. Not all ER's have radios. This particular ER was not a Trauma Center and had never, to my knowledge, received a helicopter. We only had a helipad because we would occasionally send out a helicopter.

This helicopter lands and it's an 11-month-old girl complete with ribbon in her hair who was stone cold dead coming off the chopper. The normally extremely professional flight crew was visibly frayed at the edges. They dropped onto our helipad because it was 20 miles closer than the pediatric trauma center which by air is only 5 minutes but that five minutes was important. They had been actively doing CPR on this baby since they left the baby's house so we're talking probably 45 minutes of active CPR by the time they reached us. I was assigned to the trauma room that night, so the baby was technically my patient. Yes, every ER has what they designate as a trauma room even though it is not a trauma center. That just means that it's a little bit bigger room and it has more than the usual supplies in the room.

Because Pediatrics have never been my strong point and we had a couple of nurses there for whom Pediatrics was their strong point, I basically designated myself to what I would call, a floater. I pulled meds and other things out of the crash cart. I did a little bit of everything, but nothing really hands on. In the process, I was able to stand back and see the big picture. That person that stands back and watches the big picture will often catch miscommunication between Adrenaline amped team members which can be quite helpful in itself. At least that's how I see it.

We did something we rarely do in a code. We used every single Epi (epinephrine) and Atropine in that crash cart and then we went and took every single drug out of the Pyxis. Pyxis is a name brand for our computerized drug cabinet. Pretty much every floor in every hospital uses one and most people call it the pyxis even when it's a different brand.

As this nightmare progressed, I noticed the baby's ears were a funny shade of yellow like a lima bean yellow but in various shades. I didn't really get it at the time, but I figured out later that they were old bruises on top of bruises. There was also new purple bruising around her neck in a broken thin line. That didn't click in my adrenaline-soaked mind at the time either. Afterwards we found out from Cops that they had arrested the baby's mother's boyfriend for strangling the baby which explained the purple bruising on her neck.

The guy's story to the cops was that her t-shirt was too tight, that's how he tried to explain the bruising around her neck. That made me really mad remembering the old bruises to her ears and wondering how much abuse a defenseless 11-month-old can take. The mother cared so much that she never even showed up at the hospital.

We never got that baby back as you might have figured out by now. I just had to take multiple breaks typing this story, it's still hard to relive it. To this day I remember that entire episode vividly. I remember the dress that she was wearing, the ribbon in her hair, and most of the staff that were in that room. I remember feeling stunned. I can count the times in my entire career that I cried after a code on one or two fingers. This was the worst. This was also the one and only time I have ever seen the entire ER staff outside on the sidewalk trying to cope while leaving maybe one nurse in a department full of patients. There was not a person in that room, or standing outside that room watching, who had not been operating on 110% adrenalin for over an hour. I don't know how cops or EMS crews can deal with situations like this at ground zero without beating the offender to death.

I won't say that that was the worst code I was ever in because there are too many different criteria you could use to measure that. I will say; however, it was by far the most emotional code I've ever been in.

GHB
New Year's Eve
Vegas

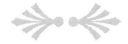

IT WAS NEW Year's Eve 2004, the end of 2003. I had only been working in Vegas for maybe two or three months. I was working at Spring Valley Hospital In a neighborhood called Spring Valley, surprisingly. It was approximately a 30 or 35 bed ER and I had an empty bed which can be a bad thing. In comes and ambulance with Ken and Barbie. Ken was unconscious on the ambulance gurney and Barbie was following along. I can see them coming from all the way across the ER and I thought oh great Barbie looks like a stuck-up bitch. As it turns out, Barbie is not only a completely down-to-earth really awesome person she is the most stunningly good-looking female I may have ever met in my life. And it did not help that she was wearing the shortest skirt I've ever seen anyone wear in public that was not a stripper. I had a really hard time paying attention to Ken who was unconscious on the gurney.

Of course, it's New Year's Eve so Ken had to be covered from head to toe in vomit, what a joy. As I'm trying to get Ken out of his vomit-soaked clothes Barbie told me just cut it off. Cut everything, she said. Well I wasn't going to cut everything because they look like really nice clothes. Don't get me wrong I'm not above cutting clothes off if you come in acting like an ass. That's just the way it works in Vegas. I'm not ashamed to admit I have even cut people's loafers and belts off. You have to be a grade A, level 10 ass to get that treatment, but it is on the menu.

I looked at Barbie and said, "really, are you sure?". That is when she explained the story. They were from Minnesota or Wisconsin or somewhere up there. They had saved their money for this Vegas trip for the entire year. Ken had spent over $2,000 between his shirts his pants and his shoes and his belt. Barbie said absolutely yes cut everything off, I am really pissed at him. By this time, I have the utmost respect for Barbie, but I am going to continue calling her Barbie because I cannot remember her name, but I do remember that she was flat-out gorgeous, intelligent, very well spoken and totally down to earth. She was in her mid or late 30s, but she could have just done a Playboy centerfold shoot the day before, I swear.

So anyway, the rest of her story was that they were at a club, an expensive club. Ken and Barbie were happily dancing when Ken started talking to some random guy and got all secretive. A few minutes later he had a small vile in his hand and disappeared into the bathroom. Five minutes later he came out of the bathroom acting like he was high. 30 minutes after that he was passed out on the Dance Floor. The ambulance crew said they figured he must have done GHB because of how she described the vile and his respirations were six per minute. Fewer than 10 respirations per minute is a pretty dangerous situation. I had never had a patient that had taken GHB before, but the ambulance crew said it was a huge thing in Las Vegas and most people that take it end up being intubated. I took their word for it. I don't remember doing much for Ken other than putting an IV and drawing blood and giving him IV fluid. A few hours later he was awake. Maybe it was less than a few hours. The whole time he was unconscious I was talking to his wife and trying really hard not to stare.

When he woke up his respirations were normal, and his Labs were negative for any problems or drugs. GHB does not show up in a urine sample or at least it did not at that lab. Ken was one lucky dude to have lived through that from what I heard about GHB. Apparently, I got to Las Vegas at the end of the GHB craze because that was the only GHB patient I have ever had. I really wonder if Ken and Barbie ended up divorced because she ultimately told me they had spent many many thousands of dollars on this trip and Ken did not even make it to midnight. Needless to say, she was one very unhappy wife.

Beware the Truth Serum

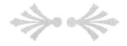

I CAN'T FOR the life of me remember where or when this happened. A husband and wife came into the ER together. The husband had injured himself somehow doing something that husbands do that wives laugh at you for. It's difficult to admit, being a male, but males do some really stupid things. I have never done anything stupid, of course, but most males have. In this case he had dislocated or broken something. A knee, a shoulder, a wrist I don't remember. The guy was not really in severe pain and he and his wife were kind of joking which is always nice. It beats having people scream in pain because we feel bad about that, we really do. This was a case where the doctor had to either put a ball back in the socket or set a broken bone, I don't recall which, but it called for what we call conscious sedation. Nowadays we've had to change the terminology to moderate sedation but that's a whole nother story. Same procedure different term. According to some government agency the different term makes it a safer procedure.

    I still remember where everyone was standing in the room. I pushed the medication into the IV that sent the guy into la-la land. I honestly can't remember for sure what the medication was, but I think it was Versed. A couple of minutes after I gave it the doctor said to the wife, jokingly, if there is anything you want to ask him this drug acts as a truth serum. Well of course the wife took it seriously. She thought about it for a minute and she asked him, "have you ever had sex with my sister?". He had to think about it for a minute, more because of his stupor then not remembering, before he responded "Yes".

    She left the room and did not come back. An hour and a half or so later I discharged him, and I never did see the wife again.

Harley Dude

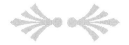

THIS WAS BACK in the trauma center that I worked at in New Hampshire. A guy about 40 years old, Give or take, was riding his Harley. He said he was only going maybe 20 to 30 miles an hour because he was riding on a residential street. Happily riding along on a warm sunny summer day, when a Ford pickup truck backed out of its driveway with the tailgate down. Our Harley Rider did not have time to stop, the best he could do was swerve hoping to get around it. He did not make it. His right foot somehow hit the tailgate. It doesn't seem like it would match up, but it did.

His right foot I want to say from just above the ankle to his toes was shaped like an s. A capital S. A capital bold **S**. We did not need an x-ray to know his foot was all kinds of messed up. Of course, we still needed to do an x-ray so the doc would know exactly which way to bend and twist to hopefully make him look like a normal person again. I pulled my scissors out and was about to start cutting his boot off when he yelled "no don't". I stopped and looked at him and he said, "please don't cut my boot off".

I just continue to look at him because I didn't think any explanation was necessary, it was obvious the boot needed to come off. He continued on at that point and said he had just bought the boots a couple of days ago and they were really expensive. They were the black shiny leather riding boots that come halfway up your calf so I could certainly understand that they were expensive.

We put an IV in him and gave him some morphine and pulled his boot off. He showed me some grimaces that I had never seen before. I have to hand it to him though, he never yelled or cried or moaned or swore. He left an hour or two later a happy guy on crutches.

Hospital Security

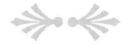

THIS IS KIND of a funny story at least it was pretty funny to me. Some years ago, before I was even working in an ER, I was traveling the country with a girlfriend who was an ICU nurse. We were working for a company call Nursefinders who did local Staffing. The great thing about Nursefinders was that we didn't have to fill out a new file every place we went, they would electronically transmit our file from city-to-city and state-to-state.

This story happens in Richmond Virginia. I ended up in some small or medium-sized Hospital somewhere in the city I don't remember where. As it sometimes happens with local staffing, I was canceled early in the shift sometime around midnight. So instead of going back to the hotel room because I had slept the entire day, I went to the hospital where my girlfriend was working. She was in a big hospital, probably the biggest in the city I'm guessing. She was working in the ICU and I did not want to call her and ask her to come let me in the hospital. I thought I would surprise her. But this is after midnight when all hospitals are locked down after 9:00 usually so I was faced with the dilemma of how to get in the hospital. Well because I was a smoker, I knew that every hospital had an outdoor smoking area, so I drove around the building until I found it. I parked near the smoking area and I wandered over and sat down with the smokers. Bear in mind that I am still wearing scrubs, so I blended right in.

When 2 or 3 smokers got up to walk back in the hospital I casually got up and walked in the hospital with them. Simple. Using signs that every hospital has I was able to fairly easily find the ICU which was on a higher floor. I'm sitting there with my girlfriend and her co-workers and somebody says, "I'm hungry". Long story short, there was no food and I spoke up and said you know every med-surg floor, typically, has sandwiches in their refrigerator for patients that did not get a meal from the cafeteria. And just like that I was nominated to go get food for multiple ICU nurses.

As a little bit of background, hospital security had been a big focus nationwide for quite some time by then. In fact, I had sat through some orientation classes that devoted a full 30 minutes to stressing that we should always ask people to identify themselves if they are not wearing a badge and it is after hours. It did not even occur to me at that point that I was not wearing a badge because I did not work in that hospital and did not have a badge. I had left my badge from the other Hospital in my car which I might have used if I flipped it around backwards to fool anyone because badges often flip around backwards on their own anyway.

I don't remember if I had a stethoscope around my neck at the time or not, I imagine probably not because there would have been absolutely no reason for it. However, it would have added to the play act. Once again following signs in the hallways I wandered the hospital until I found a med-surg floor and going by my expectations based on typical layout I found their patient kitchen. As expected, there were plenty of sandwiches, so I started loading up. In the middle of my Heist one of the staff members from the floor walks in and says, "what are you doing". Well naturally I replied I'm getting sandwiches for the ICU. I didn't think that I needed to tell him that they were for the nurses and not the patients. I was concerned however, that it would occur to him that 95%, or more, of patients in an ICU are not eating for various reasons not the least of which is that they are in a medically-induced coma on a ventilator.

Well he was fine with my story so off I go with so many sandwiches I had to push the doors open with my hip. Walking down the hallway I can see two security guards coming in my direction which is exactly when it occurred to me that I was not wearing a badge. I met up with the security guards just about the same time I came to a double steel door in the middle of the hallway. Well those nice security guards opened that door and held it for me so that I could get through without dropping any sandwiches. And that is exactly how not to provide security in a hospital. On the other hand, it's exactly how to sneak around a hospital, just act confident and wear a scrub shirt.

Another Quick Security Story

I WAS WORKING a strike back in 1999 I believe, or it might have been in 2000, somewhere in New York. I will not say where because I don't want to embarrass anyone. I was working on a long-term vent floor which was weird as I've never seen such a floor in a hospital before that or since then. I will never forget this. I was sitting next to my coworker who was also a strike nurse. I was roughly 39 years old maybe 40 years old at the time and she was well into her 50s and she was black, I am not black. Bear with me, this relates to the story. She was also apparently an ordained minister of some kind. I remember this particular night we were sitting there, and she was telling me that someday I would find Jesus to which I responded well he must know my cell phone number so why doesn't he find me? I was being a smart-ass.

Anyway, in the middle of that conversation I realize that one of the narcotics that I needed for one of my patients was out of stock on the floor. I have to go pick it up from the pharmacy. I'm not just picking up one dose I'm picking up multiple doses to get through until sometime the next day when the pharmacy normally restocks. When I called Pharmacy and told them what I needed they said an RN has to come pick it up, sign for it and show ID. They could not put it through the tube system because it was a narcotic.

Because I was still in smart ass mode after the conversation with my coworker, I asked her if I could use her badge. A minute later, off I go wearing her badge on my shirt showing a photo of a black female in her 50s while my badge was in my pocket. When I got to the heavily secured bulletproof glass looking window of the pharmacy, the person looked at my face then glanced at my badge and they shoved the narcotics under the glass along with the paper that I needed to sign. A minute later, off I went with a fistful of Narcotics.

In case you're thinking of trying this at home, it won't work. Step 1 of this whole scam was that I was able to call from an internal phone number and give a current patients name which the pharmacist could verify on computer was prescribed this particular narcotic.

Oh Shit, Did I Just Do That?

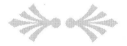

THIS IS ANOTHER non-ER story, but I thought it was appropriate. I was a new grad at Highland Hospital in Rochester New York on the 7th floor. At the time this was strictly a medical floor. I don't know if this came about because of personal instinct or because patient safety is so drummed into us starting from the first day of college. In 1993 HIV and AIDS were just becoming well known. I had worked on this floor as a tech for a full year prior to graduating and had not seen any HIV patients during that time. Now that I was a new grad, I was seeing our first HIV positive patients. I can only remember three or maybe four patients during my first year as a new grad but two of them stand out in my mind. The first one was a guy in his mid-twenties with the HIV version of brain cancer. If I remember correctly it was called Kaposi Sarcoma. The end result of this particular cancer was just what you might expect I suppose. Complete loss of memory and confusion.

The first guy I remember, I still remember which room he was in, had hand drawn pictures all around his bed from his young kids. The saddest thing in the world was his young kids, I'm guessing 5 to 8 years old, would come in to visit him and he had absolutely no idea who they were or who his wife was. That was really hard to watch.

This story, however, is about another full-blown AIDS guy in his mid-twenties. He was at the other end of the hallway all the way down on the left, I can still remember that room as well. He had a triple lumen in his right subclavian. That means a central line which is main line venous access. We could draw blood from it or we could give him massive doses of fluid very rapidly. We're talking one of the biggest veins in your body. He also had Kaposi Sarcoma. One-night working 11p to 7a I walked down to his room and I don't even remember why. When I opened his door, I saw him standing at the foot of his bed literally in the middle of a lake of blood on the floor. My first instinct was to run in and grab him so that he didn't slip and fall, which I did. immediately after performing that grand gesture it occurred to me, oh shit, now I have HIV positive blood on both hands and all over my shoes. Not that it mattered on my shoes, but it was pretty spooky, nonetheless.

My memory of what happened after that is a bit fuzzy, but I think he died that night, no doubt from loss of blood.

Suicide Attempt because of a Phone

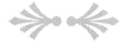

THIS HAPPENED IN a medium-sized Hospital somewhere in Nevada. It was roughly a 35 Bed ER. She was not my patient but she was in the room next to one of my rooms and so I heard the whole story throughout the night. She was 14 or 15 years old, 15 I believe. The story is that her father punished her for something or another by taking away the phone in her bedroom. This was back when cell phones were not quite as widespread as they are now and certainly kids did not have cell phones, so this was actually a landline telephone in her bedroom.

Not to be outdone in terms of punishment this girl decided she would take an entire bottle of Tylenol to punish her father. After most of a shift in the ER sucking down Mucomyst, which smells like rotten eggs, that is the antidote for Tylenol her liver enzymes were still way out of whack. I have no clue whether she had a chance of normalizing her liver enzymes over time but the word around the ER was that she was probably headed for the liver transplant list.

Another Teen Suicide

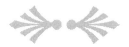

THIS ALSO HAPPENED somewhere in Nevada and no I'm not saying that teen suicides are more prevalent in Nevada. I think this one was 16 and her parents informed her that she was not going to a party that she insisted on going to. She too decided that she would punish her parents for that poor decision they made. Her younger sibling found her hanging by the neck in her bedroom closet.

  She came to the hospital by ambulance with CPR in progress. We could tell by looking that she was already gone but we worked her anyway. We worked that code with everything we had for at least an hour in addition to the time that EMS had already put in. Her parents watched from a few feet away in the doorway. I don't think she had any idea what the ramifications of her actions would actually be. I don't think she set out to commit suicide, but I guess she did teach her parents a lesson. I'm just not sure what that lesson was. That was in my top five hardest codes.

Kind of an Ethics Question

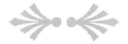

THIS CAME UP on the job a number of years ago. The hospital I was working in, and I can't remember where it was, started this conversation. I think the conversation started because someone was trying to institute a policy to cover a situation that had come up. The question is, should family members be allowed to witness a code. My immediate reaction to that question was hell no. And the reason at the time for saying that was that a code situation is chaotic enough as it is, to have screaming family members would only multiply the chaos. I will say that a code is organized chaos, but it is still chaos. I have also seen where a family member in the middle of a code situation would run in the room to the family member on the bed hugging them or grabbing them or screaming or whatever. Really not helpful. Really really not helpful.

I don't know if that policy ever got instituted and as far as I know no other hospital that I've worked at even has a policy to cover that situation. But having thought about that off and on over the years I think I have a more informed opinion now.

Here's the downside of having family member watching a code.

1) It's traumatic for the family member. Do you really want your last visual memory of that family member to be them naked, blue in color, and having their ribs broken by CPR while multiple tubes are being inserted?

2) Adding to the chaos to a point that they are a serious distraction to the people trying to do their job.

That's really the only two things that I can think of that are negatives to that situation. And now the positives.

1) At least in theory, the family member witnessing the code will never lose sleep wondering if enough was done.

2) This sounds selfish but it may prevent lawsuits against the hospital and the people in-

volved if people could see what we actually do.

3) The family member chosen to be the witness, because we can't have multiple family members there, would be able to explain to the rest of the family what they saw done.

In summary, I think it's a very good idea. However, I think that one member of the ER staff needs to be assigned to standing with that family member. The assigned escort would be responsible for preventing the family member from adding to the chaos in any way and also be there to explain what was happening and answer questions. That's my story and I'm sticking to it. I would love to hear comments or anecdotes from others on this topic.

Grapefruit as a Foreign Object

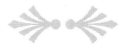

YOU MAY HAVE heard stories of foreign objects stuck inside people as result of crazy sex. I have certainly heard some stories. The most spectacular one I think that I have heard was about live gerbils inserted rectally. I have no idea how one would even accomplish that but apparently, it's a real thing.

This one happened somewhere in Florida and lucky for me I did not have to be involved but I certainly heard about it. Her story was that she was doing yoga, naked, over a fruit bowl. At midnight. Take a minute to let that sink in. The grapefruit was not inserted rectally. I will leave you to figure out the rest.

A Human Interest Story

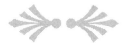

I WANTED TO include this little story because I think it's very interesting. Back in the mid-90s I was doing home health care in Florida. The vast majority of the patients were of an average age of 70 through 85 maybe 65 through 85. Obviously, they were all retired. Most of these people I would see multiple times through multiple visits but always on the first visit I would ask them the same question just for my own curiosity. I would ask them what they did for a living.

Now if you ask someone that today they would tell you I was a chef, I was a machinist, a nurse, auto mechanic, or whatever. When I asked people in the 90s who had retired in the 70s or even the 80s their answer was where they worked. They didn't tell me what they did they told me who they worked for. I would have to ask them a second time "yes but what did you do"? the answer was always oh I worked for General Railway signal or general electric or Rochester products or General Motors. But they never told me what they actually did. It was almost like they didn't understand the question.

To me that's very interesting because it tells me that they identified with who they worked for. It was like they considered it part of who they were, part of their own personal identity. Such was the employer-employee relationship based on loyalty back then. What is the level of loyalty between employee and employer now? I remember watching a movie years ago that was about a corporate Raider trying to buy a company that was cash-rich. His plan was to break the company up and make a profit. And as part of that story line I remember the management of that company was bending over backwards, even to the point of losing money, to avoid leaving their employees unemployed.

At the same time people of that era would work for the same company for their entire adult life and then retire. My own parents called me a loser because I had no interest in working for a factory for my entire adult life. I'm not sure what has changed over the years. I'm sure you could make many different arguments, but I just thought that was an interesting fact of life.

DEA Agent in Vegas

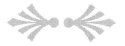

I WILL SAY where this happened because I don't think it has any chance of embarrassing anyone. This happened at UMC, University Medical Center, in Las Vegas. The only level 1 Trauma Center in the state of Nevada. There is another Trauma Center in Las Vegas but it's a level 2 and there's also a level 2 Trauma Center in Reno. UMC has the only Burn Center in the state too. I met three or four DEA agents while I was there for a year, they had some interesting stories.

This one brought in a prisoner who he was convinced was hiding balloons full of heroin in his stomach. So, the plan was we were to give him GoLytely and a commode. GoLytely came as a gallon of clear liquid that you would drink. I don't think it tasted great, but I don't think it tasted horrendous either, I never tried it personally. We normally used it for patients that were scheduled for colonoscopies or some other type of procedure involving the colon. The idea was to clean the colon out and GoLytely works very well, there was nothing lightly about it.

I was kind of wondering in the back of my head the whole time this prisoner was drinking it if the DEA guy planned on doing the digging through the commode. Within an hour or 2 he filled that commode with liquid stool. And the part of the ER that he was in was nothing but curtains between all the rooms so the entire pod knew that he had filled that commode. The DEA guy tells me to dig through it. I looked at him and said "ain't happening". Mr. DEA was pissed. I'm not sure if he went and talked to my charge nurse or not but he never tried to push the issue and I never saw him put gloves on and go through it either. As far as I know he took that prisoner and left without ever going through that commode.

Screw that, I don't even believe in the drug war.

Males are the Biggest Whiners

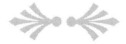

I AM A male. I will not pretend to have the level of pain tolerance to be able to Bear children. I will not even pretend to have the level of pain tolerance to tolerate a mammogram. However, I do not consider myself to be a whiner. When I have a cold or flu symptoms, I deal with it. I do not need to be waited on and I damn sure don't need to go to the emergency room with the sniffles.

What's saddens me deeply is that 80 to 90% of the people that come to the ER with ridiculous whiny complaints such as sniffles are males aged 18 to 35, give or take. Now those numbers are my own personal observations they're not official statistics and there is no official diagnosis of Sniffles. Those numbers also do not include parents who bring kids in with sniffles which is a whole nother topic of conversation.

With that being said, my God males are freaking babies. It's embarrassing to be a male. What makes it even worse is that a lot of times it's a married male who can't even manage to drive himself to the ER, so he drags his wife along to drive which means they also have to wake up the kids at 2 in the morning. All so he can be told he has a virus and should go home and suck it up. I realize that I am not seeing a large percentage of the male population. I make these statements based on the fact that the whiners that come in with the sniffles are always male never female.

In fact, I have known many males over the years who will get serious injuries and wrap it with duct tape rather than go seek help. I'm one of them. I think I learned it from my father when I was 12 years old. I was working on a motorcycle in the basement because it was winter time. Somehow, I had caught my finger in something and tore the tip of the finger so bad that had I gone to the ER I would have definitely gotten stitches. It was bleeding and I could not stop the bleeding. I wasn't crying because it wasn't all that painful, but the bleeding was scaring me being a twelve-year-old. When I went upstairs dripping blood my father's response to me was always keep a coffee can of gas next to you when you're working so if you cut yourself you can stick your finger in the gas. His logic was that it not only stops the bleeding, but it kills any bacteria.

I actually used his method sometime after that and I cannot speak to killing bacteria, but it really did stop the bleeding long enough to put a piece of paper towel on it and wrap it with duct tape. My father was an Ironman at least in my eyes. I did not much get along with him, but I did respect him. He was an engineer of some kind and worked in a power plant where there were gigantic boilers producing electricity. One night one of those boilers blew up leaving him with second-degree burns over the majority of his body. Of course, he went to the emergency room via ambulance and the doctor in the emergency room told him that he would definitely never work again, and he may or may not ever walk again. That morning when I woke up, there he was sitting at the kitchen table drinking a beer and reading the newspaper, like he always did after a night shift, only this time he was covered from head to foot in bandages. Apparently, he had said screw this and checked himself out of the ER and drove home.

He was back to work the following Monday, and this is perhaps why I have a hard time tolerating men with sniffles.

Speaking of Burns

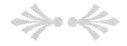

THIS HAPPENED SOMEWHERE in New York. It was a medium-sized town and the hospital was basically right in the middle of the town. The hospital was surrounded mostly by retail stores and houses. I was out in the parking lot smoking one night about eight or nine. It was summer so it was still daylight, somewhat. While I was out there, I started hearing sirens so I naturally looked around and at the same time I could see smoke rising about a half a mile from the hospital. The area of the smoke was coming from and size of the cloud could only have been caused by a house fire. I went back inside and gave my co-workers a heads up that something was going on that would probably affect us.

Sure enough, within 15 minutes or so we got a call giving us a heads up that there were going to be multiple victims of a house fire. I'm not sure if the call came from police or fire or EMS or what. We had no idea how many victims there were going to be. There were a lot of houses in the area that had two or three or four units in one house so there could easily have been up to 20 people or more in a single house fire as a worst-case scenario. We started calling in all the help we could get. We had one or two extra Doctors show up which was wonderful considering this ER only staffed one Dr. One of the doctors that showed up to help was a pediatrician which was an extra bonus.

It turned out we only got two victims from this fire, I was only involved in one of them, but it was the worst one. I don't recall if those were the only victims or if other victims got flown by helicopter to a Trauma Center. I was assigned to the trauma room that night. Again, when a non-trauma center ER labels one or two of their rooms as trauma rooms it doesn't mean that we're set up for traumas it just means that that room is probably bigger and has more supplies available within Reach. This one was a pretty big room and was pretty well equipped too.

This black kid rolls in on an ambulance gurney, without parents, that I would guess was 6 or 8 years old. I had no idea where his parents were, and it really did not matter at that point. Because we had plenty of help each nurse had a spot picked out at the bedside to do whatever task it was that you could do from that spot. I had the kids left arm, another nurse had the kids' right arm, a couple more nurses were standing at his feet and there were two doctors in the room. The ER doctor, that was normally good at his job, stood there Frozen with tears on his face. The non-ER doctor in the room with him, who happened to be a pediatrician I think, had to snap him out of it. This kid was about the same age as one of the doc's kids.

My first task was to put an IV in his arm so that we could start giving him massive volumes of fluid which is what you would normally do with a burn patient. As I'm rubbing his arm with an alcohol swab, I noticed two things. One was that he was not a black kid even though every square inch of his body was black, he was a white kid. Not that it mattered but it amazed everyone in the room that he could be so uniformly covered in soot that didn't look like soot. The second thing I noticed immediately was that his arm was severely contracted at the elbow. The biggest and most easily accessible vein in the arm is right in the crook of the elbow but I could not straighten his arm out for access to that area. I'm finding it hard to explain contracted. Imagine you pulled your arm up so that your forearm was touching your bicep and then locked your muscles so that nobody could pull your arm out straight. Except they're not doing it on purpose. In the case of this kid he had literally been cooked. He had no visible burns, but he must have been exposed to enough heat or for a long enough period of time that his tissue was literally cooked. Think of putting a turkey in the oven. Before you put that turkey in the oven you can stretch out the wings just the same as the turkey could when he was alive. When you take that turkey out of the oven, you're not stretching those wings out at all. It was the exact same case with this kid's arm.

As soon as I realized what the situation was, and that there was no way I was going to get IV access, I called out for an IO. An IO is an Intraosseous access point that allows us to give fluid. An IO needle is a specially made thick and heavy needle with a drill bit like spiral on the end of it that's made to literally drill into a bone. There are a few places we can place them but the most popular is just below the knee by a couple of inches. Just a few years ago we had to put them in by hand which was pretty hard. Now they make a little drill that does it for us.

We did successfully obtain IO access and we did give the kid fluid. We also did some CPR and we gave him some epinephrine. His heart was not beating when he got there, and we did not make it any better. I stood there at bedside thinking to myself that had we brought that kid back we would not have been doing him any favors. A lot of people would probably think that's a really cold way of looking at things.

One thing this job has done for me is it has forced me to look at life in strictly practical terms. That does not mean I would not have done everything in my personal power to bring that kid back and in fact everyone in that room did everything in their power to bring that kid back. But it does mean that I was just a little tiny bit glad that we did not succeed. At the same time, I put that one in my top five worst codes.

Incidentally, that same summer in that same ER we got a 16-year-old drowning victim. He too was DOA (dead on arrival) and we did not make him any better either. There was just too much downtime for him before he got to us. By down time I mean he had spent too much time not breathing even before EMS got to him much less before we got to him. Luckily, I was not assigned to the room he went to and there was enough help in there without me, so I avoided that one.

Why are Men so Stupid?

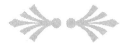

OKAY, THIS ONE is kind of funny in a sick twisted way that only an ER Nurse can appreciate. This happened in a small New York State Hospital 3 or 4 years ago. It was Christmas Eve and I'm working like I do every Christmas Eve. A guy and his wife were home with kids in bed waiting for Santa. Santa decided at midnight that it would be a great idea, while drunk, to go out in the garage and fire up the table saw while Mrs. Santa stayed inside doing Mrs. Santa stuff. Or it may have been the miter saw. At any rate, he took off about a third of his hand or went through a third of his hand. I don't remember exactly but he was likely never going to get full function of that hand back.

We had to fly him to a Trauma Center where they had a hand surgeon. Yes, there are surgeons who specialize in hands because they are so complicated. So, this begs the question how stupid you have to be to go operate power saws while you're drunk on Christmas Eve at midnight. Well I think I know the answer to that. We men are warriors, we men are builders. If we aren't busy doing important warrior and builder stuff, then what would we be bringing to the table? That's my story and I'm sticking to it.

Drug Seekers: A Huge Frustration

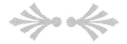

I DON'T THINK there's an ER nurse or doctor that isn't driven crazy by drug seekers. Drug Seekers are people that are addicted to narcotics and come to an emergency room with real or fake complaints trying to get narcotics. Speaking from personal observation, most of them are self-pay meaning they don't pay at all. Not only do they not pay but they often get a free cab ride home that you and I pay for. How this works is an entire conversation in itself.

Some of them are addicted to street drugs meaning heroin or cocaine or fentanyl Etc. Most of them are addicted to prescription drugs such as Vicodin, Percocet methadone Etc. Most of them seem to have no shame when they come in wanting their drugs which I suppose I can understand. How easy it is for them to get the narcotics they're looking for varies dramatically from hospital to hospital and doctor to doctor. Some doctors will give them anything they want, I think mainly just to get them out of our face. Some doctors don't want to give them anything, which I personally applaud.

They come in with all sorts of complaints from chronic pain to chest pain and everything in between. A few of the big ones are headache, back pain, and dental pain. I know a lot of people blame doctors in the healthcare industry for the fact that so many people are addicted to prescription narcotics. I say BS on that, we as a society are indoctrinated to blame others. No one takes any responsibility for themselves anymore. It seems to me like it started in the seventies or maybe it was the 80s when we blamed rock music every time some teenager went haywire. How about blaming the teenager that went haywire or possibly the parents. We want to blame the gun for every shooting but somehow, we don't blame the car for every accidental Auto death. We want to take away guns from everyone because a few people use them badly, yet we don't want to take away cars from everyone when a few people drive drunk and kill people.

I digress, I'm sorry. My point is that no one believes in personal accountability anymore.

People that are addicted to prescription drugs are addicted because they allowed themselves to become addicted, no doctor forced them to take the prescription drugs. I'd bet a week's pay that most doctors give prescriptions to get people to hell out of their office. Do many doctors over prescribe? Yes. Did that cause people to become addicted? No. People addicted themselves. Do we blame bars and alcohol manufacturers for alcoholics? No.

It seems like every night on the news we hear a story about this horrible opioid epidemic. It often sounds to me like the television news wants to blame everybody in the world except the people that became addicted. Somewhere along the line people chose to go and buy heroin and Fentanyl from a drug dealer. No one made them do it. Then when they can't afford to buy it from their dealer, or their dealer gets arrested they come to the emergency room and make up some BS story so they can get a prescription for Vicodin or Percocet. And they hope while they're there they can get a shot of morphine or a shot of Fentanyl. A lot of times they get exactly what they want and then sometimes they get nothing. But in every case, they are tying up an ER bed while somebody who really needs it is sitting in the lobby. The next time you wait for hours to get into an ER think about this. While there are a number of reasons that you might find yourself waiting in the lobby for a long time, drug Seekers are one of the two biggest issues that tie-up ER beds. The other issue is coming in the next chapter.

You are probably thinking why do we give them this stuff? Why do we allow them to tie up an ER bed for hours? The answer to that is, mostly, the federal government with some blame going to the state. Federal does not allow ER's to turn anyone away no matter what. Google EMTALA.

In addition, every time someone comes in with a complaint whether its belly pain or chest pain or back pain, we have to run all the tests to make sure it's nothing serious. If we don't and it turns out that one time in a thousand when there's actually something wrong, then the hospital and the doctor get sued. By the way this is the only country in the world that allows people to get rich and retire off lawsuits.

I know multiple people who have had 30 or more CT scans of the same part of their body per year because they come in complaining about the same chronic pain over and over looking to get drugs. In some cases, it's attention they seek, they actually need mental health care.

Another Major Frustration

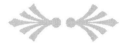

THE SEVERITY OF this varies seemingly regionally. There are, I would guess based on what I have seen and extrapolating, millions of people who use the emergency room as their main source of Health Care rather than go to a doctor's office. Now in some cases I can hardly blame them. If you just plain cannot afford to go to a doctor or to have insurance and you have a major health problem then go to the ER, nobody will blame you or think less of you.

What I have a problem with is the people who come for five, six or more times per year for a toothache or the sniffles. Parents who bring their kids in every time they have the sniffles or every time they trip and fall. Again, does no one take responsibility for themselves anymore? Can't you call your mother or your grandmother and ask her for some advice based on your child's symptoms? Or are we already at the point where every mother and every grandmother has relied on the ER for their every need and has no advice to give?

So the next time you are sitting in an ER Lobby somewhere in the United States with kidney stone pain so severe you just want to die, or a broken bone, bear in mind that it is entirely possible that 50% of the ER beds are tied up with people that should have gone to an urgent care but did not because they would have had to pay.

Suicidal Ideation in the U.S.

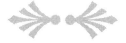

I'M NOT SAYING that we should not care, but our society has become obsessed with saving people from themselves. One small example of that would be the seat belt law. But I'm here to talk about suicidal ideation.

What that means is if you tell someone that you want to kill yourself and they call someone, you will end up in the mental health system. The front door of the mental health system is the emergency room, of course. It's really a nice thing knowing that help is out there, if someone in your family starts talking about committing suicide you want to get some help. You can't just let them go close themselves in their bedroom and hope they feel better in the morning, I get that. However, we have taken this way too far.

If you are out drinking in a bar and you jokingly say well, I might as well kill myself, or what do you want me to do kill myself, or any variation thereof you are a prime candidate to be "saved". If anyone in that bar took you seriously enough or was drunk enough to misunderstand what you said and calls 911 your whole night is shot. If anyone for any reason calls 911 and says they heard you talk about suicide, the cops will come and the cops will handcuff you and they will take you to an ER. There you will be medically cleared and then sent to a mental health facility. By medically cleared I mean we're going to draw your blood, check your urine for drugs, and we're going to do an EKG. Then we are going to take away all of your belongings including your clothes, cell phone, jewelry, wallet, purse and your shoes. We will put you some place where we can watch you and dress you either in a gown or in paper scrubs. If you resist, we will overpower you and/or get police help but you will comply in the end.

You probably think right now that I'm exaggerating. I assure you I am not. I have seen this play out in multiple states hundreds of times. You could be at a party, you could be at the mall, you don't have to be drinking in a bar. This can happen anywhere anytime. It can be a family member that makes the call, it could be a neighbor, it could be a total stranger. It could be a pissed-off spouse that knows the system. I can't count how many times I've seen that happen.

I remember one woman in particular who was brought in handcuffed by State Police to an ER in New York at 9 or 10 at night because her husband called 911. Her story, and I absolutely believed her after talking with her for over an hour, was that her husband was pissed off at her and knew the system. Her husband was a recovering alcoholic and had no job. She had the only job in the house which was delivering newspapers at night. In fact, she was supposed to go pick up her newspapers at 1 in the morning. She said if she missed that pick up, she would probably lose her job.

Her husband wanted to host a poker game with his buddies. She told him absolutely not because she knew that it was going to end in drinking. They had a fight, he called 911 and bang, she's out of the house for three days. That's the system, you can be held for up to 72 hours. She was in tears and swore up and down she was not suicidal and had never been suicidal ever. She had no record at our hospital for ever having been there for a suicidal ideation. She was not taking any antidepressant or anxiety medications. I completely believed her story. I ask the doctor if he had heard her story. He said he had. I asked him if he believed her. He said yes, he did. I asked him why he won't cut her loose because he has the right to rescind the mental health hold paperwork that the cops filled out. This particular doctor happened to also be an attorney. He did not want to take the chance that maybe she might go out and hurt herself and he would get sued for letting her go. I never did really like that guy.

The poker game lady is one case that stands out in my mind that I will never forget. However, I have seen similar situations play out more times than I can possibly count. Oh, and by the way, if this is a hospital that does not have in house mental health services (which is most of them), then they need to be sent out which often takes many hours if not a day or 2. Another bed tied up long term.

BRIAN FLEIG

Thank you for reading. I hope you liked it. I am currently working on a medical novel that I started years ago. If you'd like to connect with me, I can be found at:

Brian@Thenursinginsider.com
http://www.Thenursinginsider.com
http://Facebook.com/Nursinginsider

About the Author

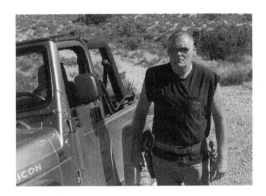

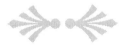

My wife was also a nurse, she graduated one year before I did. 10 months after I graduated the two of us decided we wanted to move from New York to Florida and we both took a travel assignment so that our expenses were paid. It was great because they provided us a furnished apartment so that we could get to know the area before we decided exactly where we wanted to live, and it gave us three months of paid housing to find someplace and Rent-It furnish it etc. While I was in Florida, I worked at approximately four different hospitals, 2 home health agencies and one hospice. I worked at four hospitals by doing what we call local Staffing. Local Staffing means you sign up with an agency and they orient you in the office for however many hospitals that they cover and that you choose to work in. Then when you tell them on Monday okay schedule me for Monday Wednesday and Thursday, they will book you into whichever hospitals you prefer or have the most openings. Then at 5 p.m. on your scheduled nights, assuming you work night shift, they will call you and tell you if you're going to work or if you've been canceled. It was a pretty rare thing to be canceled. If you want a week off, you just don't schedule yourself.

Four or five years later I took A travel assignment to Syracuse New York. My wife was not working by this time because of a back injury. We went to Syracuse because we wanted to visit with family and even though we were from Rochester there were no travel assignments available in Rochester. We ended up staying in Syracuse for a few years. I worked as a traveler while we lived there and that's when I started doing strike nursing. You can agree or disagree with strike nursing it doesn't really matter to me, but I loved it. That means I worked for companies that staffed a hospital with nurses while the staff nurses were on strike.

My wife and I started our own travel nurse agency at the end of 2000. At the end of 2001 my wife was diagnosed with cancer and died in October of 2002. She was 38 years old, we had been married for 19 years and 10 months.

Between moving to Syracuse and Oct of 2002 I had done numerous strikes, a couple of travel assignments, and actually spent six months taking care of a chronic ventilator patient in their home through New York State Medicaid. My main motivation for all this skipping around was I just couldn't deal with the politics of being on staff and staying in one hospital for a long period of time. It was just non-stop mandatory meetings and he said she said BS. My parents thought I was a bum because I didn't get a job in a factory after high school and work myself to death over 40 years. Plan B, according to my parents, would have been graduate nursing school at 31, which I did, then spend the next 30-40 years working in one Hospital. I would have killed myself by the end of the second or third year. I was quite happy with skipping around.

Because our travel nurse agency had actually been quite successful, I was lucky enough to not be scheduled for shifts at a job throughout her illness. I was able to take her to every medical appointment through her illness. After she died, I could not focus even on basic daily activity much less keep the business running so that closed a month later. I was lucky enough to have the money that I didn't have to work immediately but two months later I did. It had been two years since I stepped foot in a hospital and my brain was mush because of her dying but off to work I went.

In December of 2002 I Interviewed for a hospital in Syracuse which turned out to be a complete waste of time, so I took my first travel assignment since being widowed. I ended up at Queen's Hospital in Hawaii which sounds great. The truth was that I hated my life, I hated my job and I hated myself the first 2 weeks on that job. I asked myself daily "why am I here I don't belong here". Suddenly though, after two weeks it clicked, and I had the best time of my life. I spent a total of 31 days at Queen's Hospital in Hawaii. I worked 30 12-hour night shifts out of those 31 days. One of the best experiences I've ever had.

I started working in Emergency departments full-time in 2003 and that's when the real fun began. It honestly felt like starting a brand-new career and it was awesome. In 5 years of working in Las Vegas, and loving it, I did a few travel assignments in addition to working in five or six different hospitals in Las Vegas mostly through local Staffing agencies. Towards the end of that five years I got myself married again to a respiratory therapist and we ended up moving about an hour's drive out of Vegas. A year or so later we moved to Reno. A year and a half or so after that we ended up going back to Vegas, then we broke up and I ended up in Arizona.

Made in the USA
San Bernardino, CA
07 March 2019